G000123028

Bringing Mom

Back From Dementia

Bringing Mom

Back From Dementia

One Woman's Journey from Dementia to Clarity

By Susan Lake

This book is not intended to replace medical advice, or diagnose any illness, or prescribe any treatment. It is recommended that anyone seeking treatment consult with qualified physicians before embarking on any program. The author and publisher disclaim any liability for any actions taken based on the information in this book.

Bringing Mom Back From Dementia, copyright 2013 by Susan Lake. All rights reserved. No part of this book may be used or reproduced in any manner whatsoever without written permission by the author except in the case of brief quotations embodied in articles and reviews. Please address any inquiries to:
BackFromDementia@gmail.com.

First Edition
Published by Susan Lake Publications

Cover Painting – "The Tree of Renewal" by Susan Lake
Cover Photo – Bob Baldwin
Cover Design – Deb Sibony

Library of Congress
ISBN – 978-0-9893705-1-6

In loving memory of Larry Danielson

Table of Contents

Bringing Mom
BACK FROM DEMENTIA

By Susan Lake
Copyright - 2013

Preface

Cases of dementia have been increasing rapidly all over the globe. I personally went through the very bumpy roller coaster ride of my mother's dementia onset and the great relief of discovering some solutions that helped her find improvement with many of her faculties. In writing this book, I hope my direct experience will encourage people to find positive and practical solutions for dealing with dementia.

A few years ago my mother suddenly fell into an extreme form of dementia. It seemed like almost overnight she became incapable of remembering anything in her short-term memory. Her wellbeing was rapidly being compromised, and every aspect of her life was endangered. Every part of my life changed also. I was suddenly deluged with situations I hadn't been prepared for. It was hard to know where to start, as there was a general lack of public knowledge regarding improvement of dementia conditions.

The doctors I initially spoke with felt that there was

probably nothing that could be done to change my mother's course. And that also seemed to be the general belief of other people that I talked with about my mother's plight. Fortunately, I was able to find a doctor who devised a program especially for her. That program brought back much of her memory in just a few months! By staying on this program my mother spent most of her remaining years with a greatly improved quality of life.

Since that time, I've often found myself attracting people who were either dealing with similar situations with a loved one, or who were concerned about losing memory and concentration themselves. A friend suggested I write this book, since so many people are facing, or will face, these issues. Everything in this book is true, with the exception of people's names and locations, which have been changed to protect the privacy of those individuals.

I am not a doctor or licensed health care practitioner. I am not diagnosing any condition, or prescribing any medication or therapy, and I am not recommending any program. We are all unique, and have our own special needs. I am describing the steps we took which helped my mother have a better life. I am hoping, though, that you will explore situations involving dementia with an open mind and heart. It is possible that some day debilitating diseases like this will become a thing of the past.

I wish to thank my husband for his support in helping me to care for my mother and in writing this book. Special thanks to my friend Irma Wagner for suggesting I write the book and share the success we had in helping my mother improve. And I truly want to express my gratitude to Dr. C, now retired, who took the time and energy to restore memory to a woman who was very ill with dementia. Also thanks to Rikka Arnold, Bob Baldwin, Mary Lea Balsley, Ken Kosloff, Laura Fisher, Nancy Wylde, Roz Warren, Fawn Christiansen, and everyone else who helped and encouraged me to write this book.

Wishing you success in your search for positive solutions,

Susan Lake

Introduction

My mother's journey from memory loss, and cognitive confusion, back to her state of increasing clarity, had many happy outcomes. Several months into her treatment, and mostly thereafter, she experienced improved cognitive and memory function. She became physically healthier, and had more fun. She also rediscovered some of her own passions. This was a much better scenario than what she could have been facing.

Mom was diagnosed with a progressive dementia condition. She was not diagnosed with Alzheimer's. I was not sure what the difference between dementia and Alzheimer's was and looked it up. Alzheimer's is a type of dementia, but not the only type. The various types of dementia often have similar outward expressions but the causes vary from type to type.

Basically, most of my mother's short-term memory, and her self- preservation instincts had disappeared rapidly, and suddenly! The exact cause, or causes, of her dementia were not known for certain, but there were some probable contributing factors, which will be discussed in this book. From the onset of her illness, I tried to find out as much as possible about ways to help people with dementia. I looked into and studied the effects of stress, and shock on the body, especially the nervous systems and the brain, the effects of hormonal and nutritional imbalances, the benefits of relaxation, prayer, meditation, brain exercising activities, companionship, the use of special drugs, nutrition and the possibility that dementia can come through genetic tendencies. Strokes, hypothyroidism, diabetic tendencies, poor nutritional intake, circulatory problems, lack of exercise and stimulation, as well as arteriosclerosis can be contributing factors. I personally think that all of these potential causes should be looked at seriously.

In my mother's case, her increased wellbeing came about mostly through dietary, nutritional, and hormonal re-balancing. Later on, after she was doing better, new and once forgotten activities were enormously helpful to her. But first, her body needed a whole new program. As an advocate for her, I tried to hold the vision of a possible improvement. I would have been thrilled if she had been interested in meditating or relaxation, but Mom had no interest in those things. She had no interest in anything she considered unscientific. She was not interested in anything spiritually or philosophically oriented. She ended up being helped and nurtured in a way that she could accept and be comfortable with. She also had other physical problems, which were on going before the dementia became apparent, which had to be taken into consideration. Once we had a program to follow, she made amazing progress! I believe that a healthier person could do even better on their recovery pathway than she did. It is tragic when people give up too soon before they know more about the possibilities out there. But with hope, and intention, there is often progress! Now, here is my mother Laura's story.

Chapter 1 – Close To The Precipice

Dementia is a mental condition characterized by memory failures, personality changes, and impaired reasoning.

Many people believe that cognitive dysfunctions, including dementia, are hereditary. Others would say stress is the main culprit, while still others talk about unhealthy diet, lack of exercise, and lack of engaging mental activities for the mind, as the causes of dementia. Some others would point to physical problems, such as impaired circulation, and strokes as causes of dementia. In my Mother's case, I could say all of the above were probably contributing factors.

Most of my parents' family members had no mental decline even with advanced age. Many of my relatives on both sides of the family lived into their late nineties and remained mentally healthy for their whole lives. There were some exceptions in my maternal grandmother's family. Out of eight children, two did have dementia with catastrophic results that I personally witnessed.

One relative had a series of strokes and then went into a very crazed, and paranoid, form of dementia. She became so lost in her fears that she would often physically attack people because she was afraid that they were going to harm her. As a result she was placed in a nursing home and sedated for many years.

One of her sisters also suffered from dementia, which seemed to come about after many difficult shocks in her personal life. She had a much happier time than her sibling, and was living in a fairly pleasurable fantasy world. The only problem was that she had no short-term memory. She was pretty much helpless to do anything or make any decisions for herself. Someone "helping her," gave her two blank checks and asked her to sign them so they could get some groceries for her. She signed the checks without suspicion, only to have her "helper" steal twenty thousand dollars out of her bank account!

I was living out of state, and going to school, while most of these events took place. But living with these tragic events impacted my parents profoundly! When I came home for a visit, they were both very upset about witnessing the ravages of dementia. I ended up having some very bizarre conversations with both my parents.

My father seriously asked me to shoot him if he ever got "that way," and my mother made some equally peculiar requests. I remember trying to calm the conversation down with humor, "No Mom, I am not going to push you onto the ice, and Daddy, I don't think I would feel too good sticking a gun to your head! Maybe you could both shoot yourselves while jumping into an active volcano?" They weren't laughing at all at my attempts at absurd humor. Finally, I said, "Look, I will help you if something like that ever happens, but let's hope it doesn't." It didn't happen to my dad. When he did pass away, he was very cognizant up to the end. As you know, it was different with my mom. While there was some dementia in her family, there were also many other possible causes at play, which sadly, many older people experience.

One of the challenges that faced my mother was coping with the frequent deaths of many of her friends as well as dealing with the loss of my father some years before. Although my mother did have good social and conversational skills, she was very uncomfortable with the idea of going to a senior center, or taking classes, or putting herself in any situation where she didn't know the people.

Her circles of friends and acquaintances were

shrinking, and so were the sources of stimulation that she might have gotten from interacting more. She socialized less and less. In addition to her own shyness, many of her longtime friends were having physical issues of their own and could not get around as easily as before. Although we tried to compensate, she really missed being with her peers.

And she had more challenges besides growing loneliness and shyness. She developed a very pronounced form of osteoporosis. Her back was very uncomfortable and so were her knees, she experienced excruciating pain with every step.

She was starting to eat a lot more junk food, especially sugar, a guilty pleasure. She was secretly becoming a sugar addict and was hiding boxes of sweets throughout her house, so that no one would realize the extent of her consumption. Probably she was trying to give herself some pleasure, but that ended up creating some serious issues.

And that wasn't the end of the trying situations for her. Her finances were under ongoing strain, and she had a perpetual fear about not being able to care for herself.

With all of this happening, she was having issues with her thyroid gland. She had been on thyroid medication since she was a teenager. Her longtime doctor had read an article linking some forms of thyroid medication to aggravation of osteoporosis. He decided that he should cut her dosage down. At the time my mother knew that this was a very bad idea, and tried to talk him out of it but he insisted that she needed to try this. This turned out to be disastrous for her! She had been used to getting up around seven in the morning and getting on with her day. When her thyroid dosage was lowered she was exhausted most of the time, often barely dragging herself out of bed around noon. She felt tired most of the day and had a harder time focusing. She went back to her doctor to ask him to raise her thyroid level. He refused, saying she should give herself more time to try this since it had ONLY been three months! It was clear to my mom, as well as everyone around her, that this wasn't working! Yet she was resistant to getting a second opinion from another doctor.

In spite of her extreme fatigue all the time, her memory still seemed OK. Later it seemed clear that the changes in her thyroid supplement and the sluggishness that followed were contributing factors to her decline.

Chapter 2 – What Happened Next

As you can see, my mother was experiencing all kinds of stress in her life, as well as, problems with her body. She also had a lot of pride and was hesitant to talk about what was upsetting her because she didn't want to be a "complainer." Almost anyone in her situation would have felt way too pressured, but she tried to soldier through it. She was going through much more than I even realized.

A ritual of sorts had developed. Frequently we would dine with Mom at her favorite restaurant that was near her house. I had seen her recently and she seemed fine, at least mentally. She had been entertaining some houseguests; so it had been about two weeks since we had gone with her to her "hang out."

When I had seen her two weeks before she had been quite articulate and independent, which was her way. I called her to invite her to the restaurant and the conversation went like this: I said, "Hi Mom, would you like to go out for a meal this weekend?" She replied, "That sounds great! Where do you want to go?" I responded, "Well, normally you prefer to go to the Harvest Bistro, would you like to go there?" Her response really shocked me. She said, "That sound's great, where is the Harvest Bistro?" "It is right near your house Mom, on Kings Road." The next shock came when Mom said, "Where is Kings Road?" She had been driving up and down Kings Road for decades, and it was only eight blocks from her house. What had happened? I stopped what I was doing and went over there right away. What transpired next was even more of a jolt!

It had taken me about a half hour to get over to her house. When I arrived, she was glad to see me but didn't remember much about the conversation we had just had. What had happened in two weeks? How did she lose this much memory so quickly? And there was much more.

As a child of the Great Depression, she had come to believe that you should not throw away or give away anything that still might have some use. The house was always overstuffed, as far as I was concerned. Since I had last seen her, that tendency of hers to hang onto worn out things seemed to have increased exponentially!

Normally I would not go into Mom's home office out of respect for her privacy. Because my mother was behaving so strangely that day I felt like I should. Her office literally had piles of paper from the floor almost to the top of her desk. She seemed very confused, and also fearful that I would find something that she didn't want me to see. And I did! I found out that she had hit several cars recently and was being sued. (Fortunately the cars she had hit were in a parking lot and no one was in them at the time.) I also found numerous letters from the IRS asking her about a tax situation, but she hadn't responded in any way for months.

But that was not the scariest thing I found in her office. Her houseguests had filled out paperwork giving them complete access to her finances, including ownership of her house! Fortunately something stopped her from signing these papers. I then realized that there were some very predatory people in her life. I had never been comfortable with these people, but my mom had been entertaining them for decades when they traveled through her area. In spite of my discomfort I had never dreamed that they were capable of such intentional manipulation!

A friend asked me how Mom could have possibly

deteriorated so much in several weeks, without major warning signs. It is a good question.

Although I had been on the alert for a while, my mother had seemed clear and cognizant when I had seen her last. She also had been clear in our phone conversations, until the fateful conversation I just mentioned. I was later told that she might have had some very small strokes during this period, which may explain why she had deteriorated so quickly.

Because she usually was very composed in her conversation, she seemed like she was doing better than apparently she had been. It had all become too much for her, and she needed help. I was feeling very overwhelmed by the realizations flooding into my mind. I knew we needed to find some answers to her predicament quickly!

One of the promises she had extracted from me, some years before was that she could always stay in her home, if she ever became incapacitated in any way. I wanted to keep that promise to her. But clearly she wasn't safe, and support was needed to help her with her situation.

Chapter 3 – Cartoons and Scary Movies

My mother's closest friend of over forty years lived several doors from her. Paula and my mother had been neighbors and friends for much of their adult life. I really hated to bother Paula, because she had just gone through a bout with cancer, and had recently experienced multiple deaths in her family. But it was really good that we spoke, because she was very helpful and supportive.

I told Paula the whole story. Paula looked at me for a few minutes and then said, "You have a real problem on your hands! But I will talk with Laura's other friends in the neighborhood, and we will watch her more closely." This was none too soon because of what unfolded in the next few days.

I also spoke with my mom's housemate who lived in a part of my mother's home. He was often on the road with his sales work, and was frequently away for many weeks at a time, sometimes more than a month, because of his job. He would normally return to my mother's house for a few weeks and then take off again. He thought I was overreacting, at first, when I told him about my mother's rapid mental change. He was coming back in about a week, and that was some relief to me, at the time, because there would be someone in the house with her soon.

I made an appointment with her doctor of many years. This was the same person who had lowered her thyroid dosage. He couldn't see her for more than a week, even though I tried to impress upon his assistant that this was an emergency! I started to make calls to look for other doctors that might have some understanding about reversing Mom's condition. In the next few days, so much occurred.

A few days after Paula and I had spoken, she accompanied my mother to the grocery store with my mother driving. My mother couldn't remember how to drive home! Paula was as shocked as I had been several days before.

A day or two later a strange man was going around Mom's neighborhood ostensibly looking for work. Mom invited him in and proceeded to talk with him and fix him a meal. Shortly afterwards some people doing missionary work for their church knocked on Mom's door looking for souls to save. Mom invited them in and made them a meal along with the mysterious man. I guess they were having an interesting conversation. Around the time of this impromptu party, Paula got a weird feeling. She decided to go see how my mom was faring.

When she came in, she saw the man wandering around my mother's house, opening drawers and closets and going though things. It is an understatement to say that Paula was feeling terrified in his presence! The missionaries were being quite nice, but, according to Paula, they had no clue that my mother wasn't remembering anything they were telling her. I am very glad they showed up, because they may have saved my mom in ways that they weren't thinking of that day! As Paula told me later that day on the phone, she decided to "send that man away!" Apparently she glared at him and radiated disapproval until he left. Bravo Paula!

A week later, my mother's housemate was back for a few weeks. He acknowledged that she was faltering.

I went with Mom to her appointment with her doctor. It was very disappointing! I attempted to tell her doctor privately that my mother had very quickly lost a considerable amount of her memory and understanding. He said something to the effect that he thought that I was overreacting to her becoming old. In spite of her extreme fatigue, since her thyroid dosage had been lowered, he refused to give her a higher dosage. Also I felt like my mother's personality was annoying him. I wasn't even sure that he liked her. He seemed dismissive of what she told him. He was more courteous to me, but basically said that she was getting old and that we couldn't do much to change things. He was elderly himself, and I wondered if he was really listening to his own words. Would he want this sort of treatment? The one good thing that happened was that he thought she could have some hearing loss. He wrote a prescription for a hearing exam and hearing aids if she needed them.

Chapter 4 – Now Hear This!

My mother had no problem wearing her thick glasses. She used her walker when she felt she should, and didn't seem self-conscious about it, but Mom was very upset with me for suggesting she have a hearing exam! She didn't want to wear one of "those things and have people see it!" She was referring to hearing aids. I wasn't sure if she needed help with her hearing. But I had come to realize that she was well spoken enough to respond with pleasantries, even if she wasn't hearing the conversation correctly.

It was very difficult getting her to have a hearing exam, but it was worth it. It turned out that she had a small amount of hearing loss in one ear, but was nearly deaf in the other. The deaf ear wasn't causing her to forget how to drive home, but it was compounding her diminishing memory and comprehension. It is impossible to remember a conversation one has not really heard.

She received two tiny hearing aids with a real scowl on her face. Then she suddenly was hearing birds singing, cars honking, and people speaking across the room! Her frown really turned upside down, because the world of sound was opening back up to her. She was still having her problems, but was feeling better because she was hearing more. I strongly recommend that anyone with a memory problem check out their hearing also!

I knew the clock was ticking, but so far, everyone I spoke with felt that there was nothing that could be done to improve my mother's memory or cognitive function. I wanted her to be able to stay in her own home because she had made it very clear to me that she needed that for her own happiness. She had stated clearly that she did not want to lose her freedom. She also felt she would burden her kids by living in their homes, and had said so numerous times.

I had recently visited several nursing homes, "just in case," and they were depressing to me. I knew that my mother would feel terrible there. The managers of each facility I visited were very nice, but also seemed to believe that there was no hope for people in my mom's condition other than medicating them if they became too rambunctious or depressed. Suddenly a memory came up in my mind, which was the beginning of the solution for her.

Chapter 5 – Help Is On The Way

A few years before, I'd had some intravenous (I-V) chelation, (key-lay-shon), treatments for some heavy metal overload. Chelation treatments vary in size and exact content, but they are often an I-V drip used to remove heavy metals, and other toxins, from the arteries that can build up over time. It is thought to help improve circulation. There now are oral supplements that can help with the chelation process, and also there are chelation suppositories that the public can buy as well. Many people I have spoken with get very good results using these, and find them economical, and easy to work with. I wasn't aware of these other modalities when I was looking for help for my mother, but they might have been helpful to her.

When I had the chelation treatments several years before, I had always felt re-energized, a day or two after the treatments. It had been a good experience for me. I suddenly remembered that there were some people in the chelating room that claimed the treatment was helping their memories. They were experiencing better recall with increased blood flow that came from clearing the toxins from their arteries. I was wondering if chelation would help restore my mother's memory, by increasing the circulation throughout her body and her head/brain. I wanted to find a doctor that gave chelation treatments and who was very knowledgeable about thyroid.

My mother's exhaustion was very obvious, since her thyroid dosage had been decreased. It was clear that a doctor was needed who was not only an expert in thyroid but also in nutrition (since my mother's sugar habit couldn't be discounted). The right doctor would be open to a possible healing, or at least, a possible improvement for her. I wanted to discuss the possibility of giving my mother some chelation. This doctor had to be able to deal with my mother's strong personality, and also be in good communication with me. I was really hoping that Mom wouldn't need any drugs, particularly severe or addictive drugs! Hopefully, we could re-balance her body, and get things working better in a more natural way. Also I was hoping to find a physician in a nearby location, as I was getting really tired from making multiple trips each day to check on Mom, and then go back to work.

I asked many people if they knew any suitable doctors, and after awhile, some names came back through the grapevine. After several phone calls, one of the doctors called me back. I will call him Doctor C. He turned out to be the right doctor! I was more optimistic, and relieved after speaking with him because he really did seem to get the whole picture. When I asked him about chelation, he was willing to look at it as a possibility after he met with my mother. I also mentioned her severe osteoporosis, and he seemed fairly positive that he might be able to help with that also, which he did.

By the time I had spoken with Dr. C, it had been several months since I had realized what my mother's predicament was. Her life had been turned upside down and so had ours!

Mercifully, and almost magically, Mom's car stopped running almost immediately after her memory imploded. This was good, because she was a danger on the road now. It was also amazing timing, because I didn't want to shame her and tell her that she wasn't capable of driving any more.

We had to find her transportation, or drive her quite a bit, and we were working long hours. Some of her neighbors and her housemate did help when it was convenient, but we were around more. We were checking on her frequently and had stopped making weekend plans because she almost always needed some assistance.

I found a car service that catered to elderly people and was reasonably priced, with good people running it, but sometimes their schedule was booked. If she had lived in a retirement community she'd have had readily available transportation, but she had no interest in that possibility. Given her current state I knew she would be happier being near her remaining living friends, most of whom were in her neighborhood. I was hopeful that we'd get some answers and make some progress when I took her to see Dr. C for the first time.

Chapter 6 – A Stream of Light

The day came for our first appointment with Dr. C. I had to convince my mother that it was a good idea to get a second opinion regarding her thyroid. She was forgetting each conversation as soon as we had completed it. She also had come to realize that she was having a memory problem, and we talked about that, and then she would forget the conversation within two minutes. We had a lot of repetitive talks, and my nerves were getting really stretched by all of this. Still, I believed we would at least get a map of how to proceed.

I was not disappointed! Dr. C spoke with Mom at length, and then my mother would forget everything she had just told him, and repeat the story. He said, after hearing her repeat her words for about forty minutes, that, we were dealing with "progressive dementia." He also felt that raising her thyroid dosage would be very helpful to her. Although she was forgetting almost everything she was saying, she remembered that she felt better with a higher dosage of thyroid. Her first words to him were a request for help with her thyroid.

Dr. C did not believe that Mom could sit comfortably with her severe osteoporosis for the amount of time it would take for her to have a chelation treatment of the I-V type. He did, however, think a shorter I-V drip of vitamins and minerals would help her. Her osteoporosis was so notable that he wanted to run a series of tests on her that would check that condition also. He ordered a number of tests and his nurses took various samples for them right away.

He also gave her a prescription for a higher dosage of thyroid, from a porcine source. He said that the porcine thyroid had many similarities to the human thyroid, and that it would not be dangerous to her osteoporosis. He also commented that thyroid breaks up in the tissues of the body, and for that reason, he didn't feel that the blood tests on thyroid showed everything that needed to be seen. He said that it was necessary to look at the person and see if they had symptoms, and that my mom had some blatant symptoms. She had icy cold hands and feet, as well as a lot of edema in her ankles, thinning hair, and dry flaky skin. All of these conditions were often signs of Hypothyroidism, or low thyroid function, according to his observations.

Mom was delighted that she was getting a higher dosage of thyroid supplement! The doctor explained to us, and Mom seemed to understand, that she might not feel any difference for about a month. Dr. C told her that she might forget most of this conversation, but that he could probably help her with her memory and cognitive condition as soon as he got the results from the tests, which would be in about ten days.

I felt much better because we were doing something proactive to improve my mother's mental decline. Dr. C also told me that he suspected my mom had experienced some very small, undetected strokes, which had probably pushed her in the direction of the dementia.

I took my mom back to her house and helped her write some Christmas cards. As soon as we were finished and had stamped the cards, she asked me what the cards were. I could hardly wait for the test results!

Chapter 7 – The Results Are In

About two weeks after our initial appointment with Dr. C, my mother and I went back to consult with him again. Her tests revealed quite a bit of useful information. My first reaction was surprise, because her test results were so extreme, but when I thought it through, it all made perfect sense.

She was almost totally depleted in her minerals and her hormones. She also had a raging case of candidiasis. Candida Albicans is a yeast which grows in the body. When it gets overgrown it has been shown to wreak various types of havoc. Yeast infections, headaches, and intensified allergies, are some of the things that can happen, if it gets out of control. I had also heard that it can impact memory and focus. Dr. C confirmed that and said that an overgrowth can create digestive problems, neurotoxins, brain fog and fatigue.

There were strong sensitivities to yeast products, such as baked goods, as well as to sugar and milk products. Her body was needing the right kinds of supplements and foods for her particular system.

Both hormonal depletion and mineral depletion were often thought to be components in creating osteoporosis, and a lack of some of those same substances will stress brain function. Mom was suffering with both brain and skeletal problems. Now that we knew more about this, what should we do?

Dr. C spoke about the probability of my mom having poor absorption. He said that even if she had been doing everything correctly, if she wasn't absorbing enough nutrients, she still might have some of these problems. He also stated that it's common for stomach acid secretion to decline as people age which results in poorer digestion. His first suggestion was that we include enzymes and HCL (hydrochloric acid) in her program to make sure she would break down her foods and supplements correctly.

Because he suspected poor absorption, he wanted her to have twice daily smoothies with a high nutrient powder. The smoothies had a couple of teaspoons of nutritional powder blended with about 4 oz of rice milk, one for mid morning and one mid afternoon. The powder he recommended had some rice protein, minerals, and multiple vitamins, especially B vitamins. Dr. C had spoken with me about B Vitamins. He said that B vitamins are often very helpful in rectifying problems associated with dementia. In my mother's case, he thought her poor absorption might stand in the way of her thoroughly assimilating regular B Vitamin capsules or tablets. The twice-daily smoothies would put the B Complex and other nutrients into her system in a way she could more easily assimilate. Dr. C wanted to change her diet and get her off all the food she showed sensitivity to, especially foods containing yeast and sugar.

As I mentioned earlier, Mom had been ingesting a lot of sugar. She did not want to give it up! I made a search to find her sweet things that didn't have refined sugar or artificial chemical sweeteners. Dr. C felt the artificial sweeteners would add to her issues. Many people have sensitivities to the chemical, no calorie sweeteners. I did find things sweetened naturally that were safer for people with sugar issues. I found stevia, xylitol, and some fruit juice sweetened things that she seemed to tolerate well. Her biggest temptation in the future would be when she would binge on huge quantities of sugar! More will be said on that later.

Dr. C prescribed a group of bio identical hormones in small dosages. This was not the same thing as Hormone Replacement Therapy or HRT. He told me that bio identical hormones are made to duplicate the structure of human hormones. He prescribed DHEA, progesterone in a cream form, testosterone, and what he felt was a safer form of estrogen (estradiol), as well as a continuation of her thyroid prescription. He also thought that a short I-V infusion with nutrients would help her depleted system get up and running faster. The infusion had emphasis on vitamins C, B3 (Niacin), B6, and B12. We started with the I-V's once a week and then after a while once every two to three weeks. He suggested a special injection once every three weeks to help her with her osteoporosis. Last but not least, he put her on some extra mineral and antioxidant vitamins that were to be taken with her smoothies.

Dr. C felt that due to some of the imbalances in Mom's body, and probable poor absorption, that her dietary protein should be in a form that would be easy to digest. He recommended having plant-based proteins three days a week, and animal based proteins two days a week. Although eggs are animal based proteins, he felt she could eat two eggs in the morning without a lot of monitoring.

In addition to the other suggestions Dr. C made, he also mentioned that my mother's food should not be cooked in aluminum or aluminum foil. He said that many patients with various forms of dementia, had levels of aluminum that were too high. He felt that cooking with glass, ceramic, and enamel coated cast iron, would probably be a good idea. He also said that I might want to check her deodorant and make sure she wasn't using one with aluminum in it. He wasn't sure if this was a problem for her, but recommended taking these precautions to be on the safe side.

I know that this program may seem like a lot of work, but once it was organized it was relatively simple. It is a lot more work and much more painful to watch someone decline into helplessness and be without memory and cognitive function.

We created a routine where Mom avoided certain foods, took supplements with her smoothies, and for a while had a fifteen to twenty minute I-V once every week or two. For a few months I was either calling her several times each day or going over to her house, to make sure that she took her supplements and stayed on her diet. I also put reminder signs in the kitchen and her bathroom. I had organized her various supplements into small bags with AM and PM taped to the bags. I would ask her if she'd had her smoothies, which fortunately she liked, and remind her to take the appropriate bag of supplements. She would often say, "Now why am I supposed take these pills?" I would say, "Because it will help your memory." Then she would often say "OK!" and do it. Even though she had dementia, she still knew she was having some memory issues and wanted to get better.

Chapter 8 – And We Have A Winner

When we first began Dr. C's program, we didn't really know what level of improvement Mom might experience, but we were fortifying her body so her whole system would function better and be stronger.

For about two months, she would seem more energetic, and more alert after taking her smoothies or having her I-V. Then she would sink back a bit. Still, people were noticing that she was having better comprehension, when her energy was up.

We would see Dr. C about every three weeks and sometimes he would adjust her dosages. Almost exactly three months after we had started with her program, I took Mom to see Dr. C. He was asking her how she was, and she began to talk about a "bad" meal she had the night before. Someone had taken her out to dinner at a new restaurant. She described the meals, the decor in the restaurant, and what she thought was the server's rudeness. Conversations like this can be boring, but suddenly Dr. C and I said in unison, "She is remembering!" And so she was. She remembered what was on the menu, what everyone wore, and all sorts of details. Her mind would not have retained this information even a few weeks before. Just to satisfy myself, a few days later I went to the same restaurant and saw that she was remembering the menu and decor correctly. She had gotten better. The program was working!

Was she completely out of the proverbial woods yet? No, but her memory continued to improve. Her osteoporosis was stabilized, but her chin was almost level with her collarbone. Trying to drive again was not on the horizon. Even with that disappointment, she was much happier. Her memory and sense of self were improving noticeably. She was remembering most things, most of the time. It was a much better life for her and the improvement was ongoing.

Chapter 9 – Sabotage and Rescue

Mom was definitely getting better and everyone, including my mother, was seeing the improvement. Then some problems erupted.

Late one night my mother fell. She was laying face down for several hours before anyone realized she had fallen. Her housemate was sleeping at the time she fell and didn't hear her. She only had some bruises, instead of an injury more severe, which I think was due to her new healthy diet. Still, it was obvious that she needed more physical assistance than she previously had.

The subject of a caregiver came up and my mother was very upset by the idea! She didn't want anyone to "treat me like a child." She also wanted her privacy. Now that her mind was better, she had gone back to her independent ways with the exception of her driving. Her friends in the neighborhood were making an effort to see her more often, and she was not as lonely. She felt that a caregiver would be a waste of money, and also felt it could put her in jeopardy. Her aunt had been the one who unknowingly signed two checks and lost twenty thousand dollars to her caregiver, so my mother was aware of how cautious one needed to be.

She also was insistent that she wanted to remain in her own home and not live anywhere else. I wanted to honor her wishes, but I was also worried that if she kept falling she could really suffer, and her body and mind could seriously regress, or worse.

Some other problems appeared. She was starting to sneak more sugar again. I didn't want to spoil her fun, but when she ate sugar she would start losing memory and then we'd have to get her back on track.

There wasn't enough understanding from some of her friends, and relatives on the sugar issue either. It was ironic, because some of these people had diseases like diabetes and gout, which are very diet and sugar sensitive. Still these well-intended souls were not making the connection regarding how diet can affect the brain. Mom's body and mind did not do well on sugar. If she ate sugary desserts for a few days her doppelganger with dementia would start making appearances! My inner curmudgeon was pretty frustrated by the ignorance that was abounding!

Mom had another fall, not very serious, but it was enough for some in the family to insist that she try a caregiver to help her part time. I assured her that I would watch the caregiver carefully. She was not happy about this and was expressing quite a bit of anger.

But her caregiver overall was a blessing. At first my mother was unwelcoming to her, and then she began to enjoy more help and more companionship.

Catalina became my mother's caregiver. She had been a nurse, working in hospitals, before she started to work in home care. She was used to working with elderly people, who were somewhat disabled, like Mom. She got my mother into a better routine. They took walks and went for drives nearly every day. They went to the movies and out to eat several times a week, so that my mother got some new impressions. This was good for Mom's mind and body.

There was only one problem. Catalina didn't understand how important my mom's diet and supplements were either. She was used to taking very good care of elderly people who were losing their memory and abilities. She really didn't understand that we were moving away from disability and dementia, not towards it!

She was doing a great job in many ways, and I did not want to fire her. I was having a very difficult time getting Catalina to stay on my Mother's dietary program. We had many talks about this and I felt like I wasn't getting through. Finally, I asked her to go to the doctor with me and listen in.

I asked the doctor to explain the whole program and what we had been striving for. We had been trying to keep my mother in a state of lucidity, and mental awareness, as well as give her a more pleasurable life. Catalina was listening to the doctor with more openness than she had been listening to me. I had learned the program and had really tried to explain it correctly, but his explanation seemed to be what she had needed to hear. He also explained to her why Mom needed the enzymes, why the I-V drip was helpful, and all kinds of other details. After that day I asked her to come with us to all of my mother's appointments with the doctor. Catalina became much more diligent and reliable about following Mom's program.

I was very happy about this, because Mom and Catalina had bonded, and were having fun together, and I knew Mom was safer and happier with someone like Catalina being there.

Once Catalina understood the importance of Mom's program, a lot of improvement took place in my mother's life again. Catalina really liked my mom's friend Paula and would often invite her to do things with them. There was another nice addition to Mom's quality of life. Catalina encouraged Mom to explore some of her passions, which had been dormant for quite a while. This was amazing to me because my mother had really been shut down in this area for decades.

Chapter 10 – A Parallel Situation

While my mother was generally improving, my husband and I were witnessing another dementia emergency. We had a dear friend with a rapidly failing mind and memory.

Jerry and Doreen were wonderful people to know. Jerry had made a good living counseling many people. His wife Doreen was very well regarded as a trail-blazing pioneer in her particular field. They had a great relationship, and in many ways seemed ageless and timeless.

They were inspiring role models. Doreen started running miles each day when she turned sixty-five, and Jerry played tennis almost every day. They were both very positive in their outlooks, and they loved people. They often entertained their many friends, frequently cooking them gourmet meals. They took special interest in mentoring younger people, including ourselves. Both of them were very well read, and always had interesting topics to discuss. They loved to travel and took several extended vacations each year. They were quite happy and had lived this way for many years.

Jerry began to notice that his memory wasn't as good as it had been. He also started having some circulatory problems. His hands were turning a weird shade of purple! He consulted with his doctor. Jerry was told that he needed to accept getting older, and that part of aging was memory loss. The doctor also convinced Doreen that this was just the luck of the draw, and she had better accept that Jerry would be loosing his faculties. Unfortunately, she accepted this version of reality.

This was massively frustrating to Jerry. He was intensely looking for answers! He was also rapidly losing memory and concentration at this point, and would forget any hopeful information he found. After two more years, he had lost his short-term memory completely. He would constantly tell stories of things that happened in 1930, but couldn't remember what had happened five minutes before.

For several years, before and during Jerry's total memory collapse, we had suggested possibilities to Doreen and Jerry. Finally, we begged Doreen, many times, to get other opinions regarding Jerry's condition! We suggested she look into chelation, and also suggested that Jerry should be tested thoroughly. We told her about my mother's success with regaining memory, and suggested she consider seeing Dr. C or someone who had a similar type of practice.

It was a recurring nightmare! With all the fear and concern Doreen was feeling for her beloved husband, she was stuck on the opinion of their longtime doctor. The doctor had convinced her that she just had to accept Jerry's degeneration.

Jerry got worse and worse. He stopped recognizing Doreen, and often thought she was his younger brother in 1930. He was like a terribly frightened child. She became completely exhausted and depressed from taking care of him.

It was maddening to watch them suffer like this! I truly believe he could have been helped. He was much stronger physically, and much happier emotionally, than my mother had been. He had always had good health habits, unlike my mother. My mother had improved and had her memory in gear most of the time. Jerry probably would have had a lot of improvement, but a few misconceptions were blocking his path.

When Jerry passed away Doreen was completely heartbroken. She never really stopped grieving for the rest of her life. If their last years had been happier, her grief might have become gratitude for having a long and beautiful love. Instead, she felt regretful and guilty for not trying other avenues. What a sad ending for such good people!

Unfortunately, stories like this are very common. I am not suggesting that people go into any form of denial, but it is important to look for the right kind of help. We can give too much authority to one "expert." Our older years do not have to be tragedies.

As Jerry was losing his memory he would often say, "What the (expletive) is it all about and where the (expletive) did the time go?" These are good questions.

Chapter 11 – Laura's Grand Passion

Three and a half years had passed. My mother was normally lucid, with good memory, as long as she took her supplements, and stayed close to her basic diet. The only other things that would cause her to go into a withdrawal from her memory were either illness, or prolonged anxiety. If she was ill, with something stronger than a cold, she could get very unfocused. But she would not lose her awareness to the point where she was behaving like she had before Dr. C's program.

She would lose more memory if she became very worried about something or someone, and felt like she was helpless to change things. Being stressed and genuinely worried did more damage, in her case, than physical illness. In those situations, she would get vague and start forgetting things, and it would take a few days or even weeks, to get her mind functional again.

Dr. C had decided to retire from medicine, and sold his practice to a like-minded doctor, Dr. D. Dr. D was good with my mother, and continued with Dr. C's program for her. Occasionally he would make adjustments to her program, but it mainly continued as it had been.

Somehow, Catalina produced a minor miracle! My mom had been a singer and was a good pianist, but she hadn't played her piano in at least twenty years. I went over to Mom's house one day, and discovered that my mom was playing the piano and reading music, while she was singing! My mother really had a beautiful voice and showed a lot of promise as a singer and musician. Slowly she sang less and less, until that part of her seemed to disappear. But that part of her was back! Catalina had somehow talked my mother into singing and playing the piano again. It was truly wonderful! Thereafter, my mother and Catalina would frequently sing and play solos and duets. An hour or more, most days, my mother was practicing her music, and she was really enjoying it. This had been her real passion as a younger woman, and she had come back to it.

Catalina and my mother were continuing with their walks and my mom was able to walk further than she had several years before. They regularly went to the movies. Mom was having a lot of pleasurable experiences.

A few years before, Mom's knees had become so excruciatingly painful, that Dr. C had sent her to see an orthopedic physician. Her X-rays showed mostly bone on bone, and only the tiniest amount of cartilage. When Dr. C reviewed the X-rays, he added glucosamine and chondriton, as well as MSM, and some flax seed oil to Mom's diet. He told us that she might not see any improvement for at least a year, but that this should help. He did not feel that she would be able to handle knee replacement surgery, because of her other conditions.

A year later we saw the orthopedic physician again. He took new X-rays, and my Mother's cartilage had thickened! Her knees were much more comfortable than they had been before, and she continued with the additional nutritional supplements. Mom was having a more comfortable, more empowered life.

Chapter 12 – The Finishing Line

Everything moved along routinely, in a positive sense, for several more years. My mother played music, sang, went to movies, visited her favorite restaurants, and usually was doing pretty well. Her friends and neighbors were also looking out for her, and Catalina was still working with her.

When Mom was singing in her youth, she had learned some foreign languages, as part of her musical training. With repeated singing, she was recalling some of the languages she had enjoyed earlier. She especially liked speaking Italian again. She was also remembering some French and a little Russian.

One night I had a very vivid dream. In the dream, my mother's friend Paula was looking young, and beautiful, and wearing a cheerleader's outfit. I was a very small child standing in a schoolyard, looking at a school bus. Paula was running past me smiling and waving and very happy. She was getting on the school bus and she was very eager to take the bus to the next school! Once she got on the bus, she waited. In what seemed like a few minutes, I saw my mother running by, also looking like a beautiful, young woman. Mom was smiling and waving and running to the school bus. She got on the bus and sat next to Paula, they waved one more time and the bus took off.

The night of the dream, Paula was in a convalescent home, recovering from surgery. I had gone to see her a few days before and she really seemed disconnected, and very tired. At that time, my mother was still going along in her normal schedule, and seemed pretty stable.

Before my father passed away I had some vivid dreams with the same kind of feeling, as this dream about Mom and Paula. I'd had repeated dreams of my dad smiling and waving goodbye. Nine months later his spirit did leave his body, or, as some would say, he died. I felt the dream about Paula and my mother was preparing me for both of their deaths.

A month later Paula was gone. Four months later my mother suddenly became ill, and complained about feeling tired all the time. Shortly thereafter she passed away. May they enjoy their new school and I hope the bus ride was fun!

As time goes on, I'm still grateful I was able to help my mom. We found some answers that did work for her. And I have more and more questions. Older people are often viewed in a very limited way, and because of this, they frequently miss the attention and care that a younger person with an illness might receive. I feel there are a lot of possibilities for a better way of aging.

Imagine being happy and energized, focused and valued, for all your years. Decline is not mandatory! How do we want to be treated when we become older? Can we look forward to a better understanding and prevention of negative aging? How should we be treating ourselves? How should we be thinking of ourselves? Can we create a more expansive and joyful reality, rather than a shrinking, limiting one?

I believe the answer is YES!

Chapter 13 – Exploring Further

If you want to explore possibilities that may help a person with dementia symptoms, some of my experiences might be helpful to you...

When I started looking for help for my mother, it took several months to find the right assistance. At first, I mostly encountered dead ends and obstacles. Most of the people I spoke with were either uninformed, and/or skeptical about any possibility of positive change. One doctor said that it was "preposterous" to try to unravel the damage dementia does.

There were people who said I should leave my mother alone, and let her choose a course she wanted. Why bother her if she was "happy?" She was not happy and was very vulnerable. It's hard to make any choice when your memory isn't working, let alone a good choice! Even with Mom's memory loss, she could still fool people that didn't spend a lot of time around her. She had good social skills. When she was being pleasantly superficial, these same people thought she was fine. They thought I was interfering with her life. It is good to understand the difference between interference and intervention. Sometimes we need to compassionately intervene.

One can find a surprising array of reactions when seeking some new answers. This can be discouraging, but I would try not to go into discouragement. How would we want to be treated if this were happening to us? Would we want to be ignored, and possibly taken advantage of, and then sent to a nursing home, maybe for years? Or would we want some assistance and help in getting our cognitive abilities back so we could be as safe, independent, and happy as possible?

Even though most people are still uninformed, the amount of helpful information is increasing. There will be more in the future. Don't Give Up!

It seemed like an eternity until I found Dr. C, who helped my mother. In reality, it was only three months. Then it was only another three months before she was getting back to her right mind! It really didn't take that long, and helping her was worth it.

If you, or someone close to you is beginning to have some memory and/or focus issues, I would strongly encourage you to get some help and educate yourself on these matters NOW. It is normally much easier to treat a tendency than a full-blown condition! People in mid-life often joke about "senior moments." If there is a memory or focus problem, at any age, it is good to start the research. I'm not referring to an occasional lapse of memory, but to a frequent forgetfulness, or inability to focus that seems to be increasing. If my mother, who had a complicated health situation, could have as much improvement as she did, then it looks promising for others. If possible, speak to any health practitioner that you are considering working with, before you make an appointment. This will save everyone time.

It is crucial that you have good rapport with any person who is helping or treating you, or the person you are caring for. Without good communication, the situation may not improve, or could be stalled. It was very fortunate that Dr. C could also see a possible pathway for my mother getting better. It made all the difference for my mother between a terrible decline and a better life!

Believing that a better quality of life is possible is normally the first step in finding the way to manifesting that possibility as a reality. After watching Mom return to her singing and music,

I know that much of the loneliness, isolation, depression, and helplessness that can precede and accompany dementia can be replaced by an overall pattern of improvement. Let's move gladly into our future.

Chapter 14 – The Right Path For You

I don't believe that there is one plan that works for everyone who has cognitive or memory problems. Each person has their own personal history, belief system, unique circumstances, particular health considerations, as well as their own financial situation. Finding a solution that is appropriate should be done with that understanding. Because of all these particulars, I feel it is good to find a health care practitioner who is holistically inclined, and open to integrative and/or complementary medicine. Holistic means that the whole person is evaluated. Who are they? Being intuitive is very important as well as gathering knowledge in this process!

On the side of necessary caution, we can give too much authority to old pictures that we, or others hold. Too much authority can also be given to one doctor, or one expert, a belief about genetics, or anything else you can think of. Remember Doreen and Jerry?

Having said this, it is necessary to find a pathway

to improvement that starts with something the person with cognitive issues can accept. In the case of my mother, we had had enough conversations about meditation and relaxation techniques for me to know that we should not try that approach. I knew enough about her to convince her that there was nothing to lose by consulting with a different physician.

After my experience with my mother, I think finding the right health practitioner, as well as getting the hearing checked are good places to begin. If the person's hearing is impeded, then their memory will suffer by default.

Physicians that are holistically inclined usually practice integrative and/or complementary medicine. Integrative and complementary medicine are terms which imply an openness to many types of healing modalities. This would include, but not be limited to, mainstream medicine. Other possibilities such as nutrition, chelation, homeopathy, herbal remedies, acupuncture, biofeedback, structural adjustments, hypnosis, guided imagery and other methods and forms of treatment could be openly explored as possible routes to improvement.

The laws regarding what a health care practitioner

can do vary from place to place. In my mother's case, I wanted an M.D., but that does not mean that an Osteopath, a Nurse Practitioner, an Acupuncturist, a Physician's Assistant, a Chiropractor, a Nutritionist or some other well-trained health practitioner might not have the right answers for you.

Whoever you chose to work with, though, should be able to order and correctly interpret any tests that are needed. In the case of Dr. C, he felt strongly that conventional thyroid testing was often not enough, so he looked at my mother's additional symptoms. The health care practitioner must also be very observant. Whoever you work with needs to be well versed in their field, but also very intuitive about the person they are treating.

The right nutrition, absorption, hormonal balancing, and circulatory enhancement were the keys to helping my mom become more functional. Once Mom's body and mind were working more in concert, it was much easier for Mom to connect with her better self. I never imagined she would spend her final years singing and playing the piano, speaking some languages that she had learned sixty years before, and going to the movies twice a week. That was wonderful! But initially it was necessary to get her body and brain working better before we could progress.

Getting the person's mind and emotions engaged in something they find interesting can be very therapeutic. Crossword puzzles, playing Monopoly or Checkers, or some other games, which exercise the mind, are often recommended to help revive failing memories. I don't doubt that those types of games can be helpful, but in my mother's case it was something far more personal to her. Her music helped revive her more positive abilities once her body and brain were functioning better.

Stimulating a person's true interests can be a real gift to them, and help them connect more with their intelligent persona.

Also positive companionship is vital to strengthening a fragile mind. Each person's needs vary, but isolation and loneliness don't support any kind of positive improvement. In addition to that, many people start going off the "deep end" if they feel useless, or unwanted. This is a big problem for a lot of older people! If the self-esteem is plummeting, the mind often starts following suit.

In addition to enough companionship, clean and ordered surroundings can help a person with memory and concentration challenges. If a person's living situation is in too much chaos, it sets a chaotic tone, and generates feelings of overwhelm. Familiar places to find things are helpful to the person trying to regain their memory. Clutter removal or reorganization can assist the mind in focusing better, and feeling more peaceful.

I found that my mother's level of cognizance became more elevated after she watched a really interesting or humorous movie or show, or listened to some uplifting music, or did anything that engaged her mind and emotions in a positive way. Intelligent humor, or an interesting mystery, or something inspiring, can really make a person feel more alive and focused, and is also a great stress reliever. Unfortunately there are many mind-numbing influences out there. Sitting someone in front of a TV or computer, with the less intelligent input, tends to make them less functional mentally. It's important to avoid the impressions which dull us. Feeling calmer is a good thing, feeling duller is potentially dangerous.

Some of the symptoms which might be indicative of a tendency towards dementia would include increasing memory loss, repetition of phrases or sentences over and over, difficulty focusing on normal things, increasing confusion, exaggeration of the persons strongest negative traits, paranoia that is unfounded, childish behavior, lack of basic personal protection, lack of hygiene, unprovoked rages or tantrums, severe depression accompanying any of these expressions, and strange imaginings that have no connection with the person's reality.

For our own protection, we can really become aware and try to eliminate as much unnecessary stress and suffering as possible. We all can suffer habitually and mechanically, through negative programming. Avoiding toxic situations and personalities, as well as substances, is supportive to the body and mind.

If you are the advocate/caregiver for someone, it is helpful to hold the vision of the best possible solution for them in their particular circumstances. If it is a temptation for you to sacrifice your own well being for someone else, ask someone you can trust to tell you if they see you going in that direction. I believe that we can help our loved ones without harming ourselves! There is a necessary consistency in helping another. Once you have the right system, it should become much easier to keep things going in a positive direction.

While I was involved with my mother's process, I often wished for a truly progressive support group with people that were finding solutions. I know that there are support groups for people who are dealing with mental decline in loved ones. I would like to see support groups with people who are finding actual improvement in the capacities of those with dementia. If you know of such a group or groups, please let me know.

Many of the most dangerous illnesses have essentially been eradicated from the human experience. Likewise, the old belief that every mind and body must deteriorate with age may someday be seen as an ancient superstition. If we set our intention to find positive solutions, and persevere, possibilities, and answers usually start showing up. Amazing improvements are possible!

Chapter 15 – I Wish This Wasn't Important

I really wish that this chapter wasn't necessary, but I believe it is. There is serious pollution in some of our air, water, and food supplies that potentially impact us all. Some of our electrical devices can have serious effects on certain people. The proximity to some factories, power stations, construction sites, and farming areas, create real problems for those sensitive to the chemicals, fertilizers, manufacturing materials and electrical frequencies used by some manufacturers.

Mercury is just one example of something that can become toxic and can affect brain function, but there are other metals, chemicals, pesticides, molds, parasites and poisons of many varieties that could be at dangerous levels in our neighborhoods, or work environments. If there are any sudden or chronic serious health problems that arise for us or those we care for, it is prudent to check for toxicity in our water sources, air quality, and food sources, as well as our carpets, furniture, cleaning supplies, electrical appliances and substances, we work with regularly. This may be especially important if there is any kind of cognitive dysfunction.

Our brains and nervous systems can be impacted by the wrong metals and/or chemicals in dental work, cosmetics, or toothpaste. The level of sensitivity varies from person to person. Some of us have more resilience than others. Serious illness might mean there are unknown or unseen toxins too close to us.

Educating ourselves on these matters might tip the balance between a good life and a sick life. There are environmentally aware individuals, groups, and companies that can help us out if we don't know how to access things, or what to test for. It is a good idea to become more conscious of these possible factors.

Having said all this, I still feel optimistic about recovery for cognitive disease, and that a growing awareness about potential toxins will help to create a healthier world!

Chapter 16 – Making the Commitment

As stated in the beginning of this book, I am not diagnosing an illness or prescribing a course of treatment for anyone. I am writing about what helped my mother to become more lucid and have a better quality of life. In this chapter I will list the things we did which were helpful to her. Also, there will be a list of some other courses of treatment that I have heard or read about from other people that we did not try, but that could be worth some investigation. Please check with your health care practitioner to be sure that there are no contraindications for treatments that you or anyone you are interested in helping might wish to explore.

What we did...

My mom's hearing was checked and she really needed hearing aids. She had a big improvement in her comprehension after she got her hearing aids.

Her thyroid was checked and she was given a

higher potency prescription. Please remember that Dr. C was not convinced that ordinary blood work to test the thyroid was sufficient. He also relied on observing physical symptoms, which pointed to thyroid imbalances. In my mother's case, Dr. C felt that the extreme coldness of her hands and feet, her difficulty in waking up, the severe edema in her ankles, and her thinning hair, and flaky skin, were symptoms that indicated a thyroid deficiency.

Mom was tested for allergies and candidiasis, and it turned out she had a serious overgrowth of Candida Albicans, which can create memory problems. She also had some allergies, and some sensitivities to certain foods and pollens, that can influence memory and focusing faculties.

She had broad range testing and the results showed a serious lack of hormones and minerals. This was corrected by giving her daily oral and topical supplementation of the bio-identical hormones, as well as daily oral supplementation of minerals and vitamins. Dr. C stressed that Bio-Identical Hormone treatment was not the same as Hormone Replacement Therapy or HRT. We carefully monitored this treatment.

My mother's tests also showed a general depletion

of vital nutrients, and to correct this she was given small smoothies twice a day with rice milk, and a powder called All One, the rice based version. This was a high nutrient, easily absorbable, supplement. Dr. C gave her this because he suspected poor absorption in her digestive system. While she had her smoothies, she also took her mid morning and mid afternoon supplements. This helped to revitalize her.

We looked into chelation for her. Because of her osteoporosis she couldn't sit comfortably for the normal I-V chelation time, so, Dr. C created a much smaller I-V to fortify her and help her circulation. She had these treatments weekly until her strength and memory were better, and then she would have a treatment every few weeks.

Her diet was changed, omitting sugar, wheat, dairy, and yeast rich foods most of the time. She was given enzymes to help with digestion.

We removed aluminum pots, deodorant with aluminum, and got the aluminum foil out of the house. Many people with dementia, including Alzheimer's, have abnormally high aluminum content in their tests, according to Dr. C.

There was an ongoing effort to create familiar and

also new impressions for her. For example, she had a regular schedule of walking, but was frequently taken to several different parks, so she could get her own rhythm going but have some variation for stimulation.

She was encouraged to re-explore things she had been good at but hadn't done in a while. This helped her a great deal but her memory and strength had to improve before this worked.

A concerted effort was made through conversations, movies, television, and radio, to expose her to more intelligent conversation and positive impressions, to stimulate her brain, as well as her spirit.

We avoided foods that were grown or prepared with chemicals.

We were patient.

The following possibilities were not tried for my mother's situation but may be worth some research....

Many people have reported better health after removal of "silver/mercury" fillings. This could be important because mercury, and other metals found in "silver" fillings are have been reported to create problems in cognition when there is an excess.

Besides excessive amounts of aluminum, excessive amounts of iron, and also copper, have been reported being issues in some people's cognitive problems.

Checking the vision of a person has been reported to help with improvement of dementia tendencies. There are different theories about this, one of which is that if we see better, it engages the brain differently than if our vision is blocked.

It could be important to monitor the water supply/soil content/air quality.

There is research being done on coconut oil to help improve cognitive function. Some of the same research, as well as other studies indicate that diabetic tendencies can be contributing factors to cognitive decline. This includes a condition known as diabetes of the brain, yes, you read this correctly. Notable improvement in cognition for some of the people involved in these studies has been reported with a change in diet and addition of coconut oil.

Many good things have been said and written about the following supplements. We didn't use them, but some people really think these are helpful, so it might be worth some reading...many of these supplements are nature-based coming from ancient cultures with histories of good medicine ...

Gingko, gota kola, ginseng, and iboga, bocapa, mangosteen, and chlorella are just some of the remedies that show up in many articles and testimonials.

Glutathione is being reported by some as being very helpful in improving dementia tendencies.

Also, there are a number of positive reports coming from people who have used these dietary supplements ... Lypho-Spheric vitamins, DMAE, Vitamin D 3, phosphatidyl choline, phosphatidyl serine, DHA, piracetam, other nootropics, and huperzine-A, fish oils, borage oils, and co-enzyme Q10. There may be many more supplements which could hold some benefit.

Also, several people have spoken with me about their memory working better if they spend more time in a light filled room, rather than a shaded room. The quality of light is a room is often a mood influence, but it could have deeper implications.

And there may be many more possibilities that would help prevent or improve conditions of dementia.

If you have experienced anything that you think would help, please let me know. There is a need for more communication about improvement, and eventually prevention, of the various forms of dementia, and other related conditions.

Please visit my web site for possible sources of help for dementia, as well as organizaons, which could be helpful: www.backfromdementia.com.

Hopefully, very soon, and much more easily than in prior times, cognitive disorders and mind crippling diseases will become issues of the past. It might not be that difficult if enough of us look for the answers. Let's find the truth and eradicate negative aging! It is possible!

My wish is that you, the reader, will find this book to be supportive and helpful in your search for solutions.

Very Best Wishes to You and Much Success on Your Journey!